THE RHEUMATOID ARTHRITIS COOKBOOK 2024

An Extensive Handbook Covering The Comprehension, Prevention, Management, And Treatment Of Rheumatoid Arthritis.

Vanessa Meza

Table of Contents

INTRODUCTION TO RHEUMATOID ARTHRITIS 2

    A. Definition And Overview Of Rheumatoid Arthritis (Ra) 2

    B. Importance Of Addressing Ra In Modern Society 2

    C. Purpose Of The Book 2

A. DEFINITION AND OVERVIEW OF RHEUMATOID ARTHRITIS (RA): 2

B. IMPORTANCE OF ADDRESSING RA IN MODERN SOCIETY: 5

C. PURPOSE OF THE BOOK: 8

CHAPTER ONE 10

UNDERSTANDING RHEUMATOID ARTHRITIS 10

    A. The Basics Of Ra: Causes And Risk Factors 10

    B. Pathophysiology: How Ra Affects The Body 10

    C. Symptoms And Clinical Manifestations 10

    D. Diagnosis And Differential Diagnosis 10

A. THE BASICS OF RA: CAUSES AND RISK FACTORS 10

B. PATHOPHYSIOLOGY: HOW RA AFFECTS THE BODY 13

C. SYMPTOMS AND CLINICAL MANIFESTATIONS 15

D. DIAGNOSIS AND DIFFERENTIAL DIAGNOSIS 16

CHAPTER TWO 19

LIVING WITH RHEUMATOID ARTHRITIS 19

    A. Emotional And Psychological Impact 19

    B. Lifestyle Modifications For Managing Ra 19

    C. Medications And Treatment Options 19

    D. Alternative Therapies And Complementary Medicine 19

A. EMOTIONAL AND PSYCHOLOGICAL IMPACT 19
B. LIFESTYLE MODIFICATIONS FOR MANAGING RA 21
C. MEDICATIONS AND TREATMENT OPTIONS 23
D. ALTERNATIVE THERAPIES AND COMPLEMENTARY MEDICINE 25
CHAPTER THREE 27
NAVIGATING DAILY LIFE WITH RA 27
   A. Coping Strategies For Managing Pain And Fatigue 27
   B. Maintaining Mobility And Functionality 27
   C. Balancing Work, Relationships, And Self-Care 27
   D. Tips For Communicating With Healthcare Providers 27
A. COPING STRATEGIES FOR MANAGING PAIN AND FATIGUE .. 27
B. MAINTAINING MOBILITY AND FUNCTIONALITY 29
C. BALANCING WORK, RELATIONSHIPS, AND SELF-CARE 30
CHAPTER FOUR 34
EMPOWERING YOURSELF AGAINST RHEUMATOID ARTHRITIS . 34
   A. Advocating For Your Needs: Tips For Self-Advocacy 34
   B. Building A Support Network 34
   C. Engaging In Research And Clinical Trials 34
   D. Hope For The Future: Advances In Ra Treatment 34
A. ADVOCATING FOR YOUR NEEDS: TIPS FOR SELF-ADVOCACY 34
B. BUILDING A SUPPORT NETWORK 36
C. ENGAGING IN RESEARCH AND CLINICAL TRIALS 38
D. HOPE FOR THE FUTURE: ADVANCES IN RA TREATMENT 39
Top of Form 42

SPECIAL CONSIDERATIONS 42
   A. Ra And Women's Health......42
   B. Ra In Children And Adolescents......42
   C. Managing Ra In Older Adults......42
   D. Ra And Comorbidities: Understanding The Connection....42
A. RA AND WOMEN'S HEALTH......42
B. RA IN CHILDREN AND ADOLESCENTS......44
C. MANAGING RA IN OLDER ADULTS......47
D. RA AND COMORBIDITIES: UNDERSTANDING THE CONNECTION......49
BEYOND THE INDIVIDUAL: RA IN SOCIETY......53
   A. The Socioeconomic Impact Of Ra......53
   B. Accessibility And Equity In Ra Care......53
   C. Advocacy Efforts And Policy Changes......53
   D. Promoting Awareness And Education......53
A. THE SOCIOECONOMIC IMPACT OF RA......53
B. ACCESSIBILITY AND EQUITY IN RA CARE......55
C. ADVOCACY EFFORTS AND POLICY CHANGES......57
D. PROMOTING AWARENESS AND EDUCATION......58
CONCLUSION......61
   A. Recap Of Key Points......61
   B. Encouragement And Inspiration For Readers......61
   C. Call To Action: Taking Charge Of Your Ra Journey......61
   D. Looking Ahead: Hope For A Future Without Rheumatoid Arthritis......61

A. RECAP OF KEY POINTS 61
B. ENCOURAGEMENT AND INSPIRATION FOR READERS 63
C. CALL TO ACTION: TAKING CHARGE OF YOUR RA JOURNEY ... 64
D. LOOKING AHEAD: HOPE FOR A FUTURE WITHOUT RHEUMATOID ARTHRITIS 65
THE END 67

INTRODUCTION TO RHEUMATOID ARTHRITIS

A. Definition And Overview Of Rheumatoid Arthritis (Ra)

B. Importance Of Addressing Ra In Modern Society

C. Purpose Of The Book

A. DEFINITION AND OVERVIEW OF RHEUMATOID ARTHRITIS (RA):

Definition: Rheumatoid arthritis (RA) is a chronic autoimmune disease that primarily affects the joints. In RA, the immune system mistakenly attacks the body's own tissues, particularly the synovium, a thin membrane that lines the joints. This results in inflammation, pain, stiffness, and swelling in the affected joints.

Pathophysiology: The exact cause of RA is not fully understood, but it is believed to involve a combination of genetic, environmental, and hormonal factors. The immune system's abnormal response leads to the production of inflammatory chemicals, such as cytokines, which contribute to joint damage and other systemic effects.

Symptoms: The symptoms of RA can vary from person to person but commonly include joint pain, stiffness (especially in the morning or after periods of inactivity), swelling, and reduced range of motion. RA can also affect other organs and systems in the body, leading to complications such as rheumatoid nodules, cardiovascular disease, and lung involvement.

Diagnosis: Diagnosis of RA typically involves a combination of medical history, physical examination, laboratory tests (such as blood tests for inflammatory markers and autoantibodies), and imaging studies (such as X-rays and ultrasound) to assess joint damage.

Treatment: While there is no cure for RA, various treatments aim to manage symptoms, slow disease progression, and improve quality of life. Treatment approaches may include medications (such as disease-modifying antirheumatic drugs and biologic agents), physical therapy, lifestyle modifications, and in some cases, surgery to repair or replace damaged joints.

B. IMPORTANCE OF ADDRESSING RA IN MODERN SOCIETY:

Prevalence: Rheumatoid arthritis affects millions of people worldwide, making it one of the most common autoimmune diseases. Its prevalence varies across different populations and tends to be more common in women and older adults.

Impact on Quality of Life: RA can significantly impact a person's quality of life by causing chronic pain, disability, and limitations in daily activities. It can also lead to emotional and psychological challenges, such as depression and anxiety, due to its chronic nature and unpredictable course.

Economic Burden: RA imposes a substantial economic burden on individuals, families, healthcare systems, and society as a whole. The costs associated with medical care, medications, rehabilitation, and lost productivity due to work disability can be considerable.

Public Health Challenge: Addressing RA is not only important at the individual level but also at the public health level. Effective management of RA requires timely diagnosis, access to appropriate healthcare services, patient education, and public awareness campaigns to promote early intervention and optimal treatment outcomes.

C. PURPOSE OF THE BOOK:

Education and Awareness: The purpose of the book is to educate readers about rheumatoid arthritis, including its causes, symptoms, diagnosis, and treatment options. By increasing awareness and understanding of RA, the book aims to empower individuals affected by the disease, their families, caregivers, and the general public to make informed decisions about managing the condition.

Support and Guidance: In addition to providing factual information, the book may also offer practical advice, resources, and support for individuals living with RA. This could include tips for managing symptoms, coping strategies for dealing with the emotional and social impact of the disease, and guidance on navigating the healthcare system.

Advocacy and Research: Furthermore, the book may advocate for greater investment in research to advance our understanding of RA and develop more effective treatments. By highlighting the importance of addressing RA as a public health priority, the book may encourage policymakers, healthcare providers, and research institutions to prioritize efforts to improve care and outcomes for individuals with RA.

CHAPTER ONE

UNDERSTANDING RHEUMATOID ARTHRITIS

A. The Basics Of Ra: Causes And Risk Factors

B. Pathophysiology: How Ra Affects The Body

C. Symptoms And Clinical Manifestations

D. Diagnosis And Differential Diagnosis

A. THE BASICS OF RA: CAUSES AND RISK FACTORS

Causes: Rheumatoid arthritis (RA) is an autoimmune disorder, which means the body's immune system mistakenly attacks its own tissues. The exact cause of RA is not fully understood, but it is believed to result from a combination of genetic, environmental, and hormonal factors. Certain genetic variations predispose individuals to develop RA, but environmental triggers, such as smoking, infections, and hormonal changes, may also play a role in initiating the autoimmune response.

Risk Factors: Several factors can increase the risk of developing RA:

Genetics: Individuals with a family history of RA are at higher risk.

Gender: RA is more common in women than in men.

Age: While RA can occur at any age, it most commonly starts between the ages of 30 and 60.

Smoking: Smoking increases the risk of developing RA, particularly in individuals with genetic predisposition.

Obesity: Obesity is associated with an increased risk and severity of RA.

Environmental Exposures: Exposure to certain environmental factors, such as air pollution and occupational hazards, may contribute to the development of RA.

B. PATHOPHYSIOLOGY: HOW RA AFFECTS THE BODY

Autoimmune Response: In RA, the immune system mistakenly attacks the synovium, the lining of the joints, leading to inflammation and joint damage. The immune cells release inflammatory cytokines, such as tumor necrosis factor-alpha (TNF-alpha) and interleukin-1 (IL-1), which promote inflammation and tissue destruction.

Synovial Inflammation: Chronic inflammation of the synovium leads to the formation of pannus, an abnormal tissue that erodes cartilage and bone within the joint. This results in joint pain, swelling, stiffness, and eventually, deformity and loss of function.

Systemic Effects: RA is not limited to the joints; it can also affect other organs and systems in the body. Systemic manifestations of RA may include rheumatoid nodules (firm lumps under the skin), cardiovascular complications (such as increased risk of heart attack and stroke), lung involvement (such as interstitial lung disease), and systemic inflammation that affects multiple organs.

C. SYMPTOMS AND CLINICAL MANIFESTATIONS

Joint Symptoms: The hallmark symptoms of RA include joint pain, swelling, stiffness (particularly in the morning or after periods of inactivity), and reduced range of motion. RA commonly affects small joints, such as those in the hands and feet, but can also involve larger joints, such as the knees, shoulders, and hips.

Fatigue: Many individuals with RA experience fatigue, which can be debilitating and affect daily functioning.

Systemic Symptoms: In addition to joint symptoms, RA can cause systemic symptoms such as fever, weight loss, and generalized weakness.

D. DIAGNOSIS AND DIFFERENTIAL DIAGNOSIS

Clinical Evaluation: Diagnosis of RA involves a thorough medical history and physical examination by a healthcare provider. The presence of joint symptoms, along with other clinical manifestations and risk factors, may raise suspicion for RA.

Laboratory Tests: Blood tests are commonly used to support the diagnosis of RA. These may include tests for inflammatory markers such as C-reactive protein (CRP) and erythrocyte sedimentation rate (ESR), as well as tests for autoantibodies such as rheumatoid factor (RF) and anti-cyclic citrullinated peptide (anti-CCP) antibodies, which are commonly elevated in RA.

Imaging Studies: Imaging studies such as X-rays, ultrasound, and magnetic resonance imaging (MRI) may be used to assess joint damage and inflammation, particularly in cases where the diagnosis is unclear or to monitor disease progression over time.

Differential Diagnosis: RA shares symptoms with other forms of arthritis and autoimmune diseases, making differential diagnosis important. Conditions that may mimic RA include osteoarthritis, systemic lupus erythematosus (SLE), psoriatic arthritis, and infectious arthritis, among others. A comprehensive evaluation is necessary to differentiate RA from other potential causes of joint symptoms.

CHAPTER TWO

LIVING WITH RHEUMATOID ARTHRITIS

A. Emotional And Psychological Impact

B. Lifestyle Modifications For Managing Ra

C. Medications And Treatment Options

D. Alternative Therapies And Complementary Medicine

A. EMOTIONAL AND PSYCHOLOGICAL IMPACT

Chronic Stress: Living with RA can be emotionally challenging due to the chronic nature of the disease and its unpredictable course. Dealing with ongoing pain, fatigue, and disability can lead to stress, anxiety, and depression.

Social Isolation: RA may limit a person's ability to participate in social activities and maintain relationships, leading to feelings of isolation and loneliness.

Body Image Issues: Changes in physical appearance due to joint deformities or swelling may affect self-esteem and body image.

Coping Strategies: It's important for individuals with RA to develop coping strategies to manage the emotional and psychological impact of the disease. This may include seeking support from friends, family, or support groups, practicing stress-reduction techniques such as mindfulness or meditation, and seeking professional counseling if needed.

B. LIFESTYLE MODIFICATIONS FOR MANAGING RA

Regular Exercise: Exercise is an essential part of managing RA as it helps improve joint flexibility, strength, and overall physical function. Low-impact activities such as swimming, walking, yoga, and tai chi are beneficial for individuals with RA.

Healthy Diet: A balanced diet rich in fruits, vegetables, whole grains, lean proteins, and omega-3 fatty acids may help reduce inflammation and support overall health. Some individuals with RA may benefit from avoiding certain foods that trigger inflammation, such as processed foods, refined sugars, and saturated fats.

Stress Management: Managing stress is important for managing RA symptoms. Techniques such as relaxation exercises, deep breathing, and mindfulness can help reduce stress levels.

Joint Protection: Practicing joint protection techniques, such as using assistive devices, ergonomic tools, and modifying daily activities to reduce joint strain, can help preserve joint function and minimize pain.

C. MEDICATIONS AND TREATMENT OPTIONS

Disease-Modifying Antirheumatic Drugs (DMARDs): DMARDs, such as methotrexate, hydroxychloroquine, and sulfasalazine, are the cornerstone of RA treatment. These medications help suppress the underlying inflammation and slow down the progression of joint damage.

Biologic Therapies: Biologic drugs, such as tumor necrosis factor (TNF) inhibitors, interleukin-6 (IL-6) inhibitors, and B-cell inhibitors, target specific components of the immune system involved in RA inflammation. These drugs are often used in combination with DMARDs for individuals who do not respond adequately to conventional treatments.

Nonsteroidal Anti-Inflammatory Drugs (NSAIDs): NSAIDs, such as ibuprofen and naproxen, help relieve pain and reduce inflammation in RA. They are often used for short-term symptom relief.

Corticosteroids: Corticosteroids, such as prednisone, may be used to quickly reduce inflammation and relieve symptoms during disease flares. However, they are typically used at low doses and for short periods due to the risk of long-term side effects.

D. ALTERNATIVE THERAPIES AND COMPLEMENTARY MEDICINE

Acupuncture: Acupuncture involves the insertion of thin needles into specific points on the body to alleviate pain and promote healing. Some individuals with RA may find acupuncture helpful for pain relief and improving joint function.

Massage Therapy: Massage therapy can help reduce muscle tension, improve circulation, and relieve pain in individuals with RA. Gentle techniques, such as Swedish massage or lymphatic drainage, are typically used to avoid exacerbating joint inflammation.

Dietary Supplements: Some individuals with RA may use dietary supplements such as fish oil, turmeric, and ginger to help reduce inflammation and manage symptoms. However, it's important to consult with a healthcare provider before taking supplements, as they may interact with medications or have side effects.

Mind-Body Practices: Mind-body practices such as meditation, yoga, and tai chi can help reduce stress, improve mood, and enhance overall well-being in individuals with RA. These practices may also help improve joint flexibility and function.

CHAPTER THREE

NAVIGATING DAILY LIFE WITH RA

A. Coping Strategies For Managing Pain And Fatigue

B. Maintaining Mobility And Functionality

C. Balancing Work, Relationships, And Self-Care

D. Tips For Communicating With Healthcare Providers

A. COPING STRATEGIES FOR MANAGING PAIN AND FATIGUE

Pacing Activities: Break tasks into smaller, manageable chunks and alternate between periods of activity and rest to prevent overexertion and fatigue.

Use of Assistive Devices: Utilize assistive devices such as braces, splints, canes, or ergonomic tools to reduce strain on joints and conserve energy.

Heat and Cold Therapy: Applying heat packs or cold packs to affected joints can help alleviate pain and reduce inflammation.

Relaxation Techniques: Practice relaxation techniques such as deep breathing, guided imagery, or progressive muscle relaxation to reduce stress and manage pain.

Medication Management: Take prescribed medications as directed to manage pain, inflammation, and fatigue. Communicate with your healthcare provider about any concerns or side effects.

B. MAINTAINING MOBILITY AND FUNCTIONALITY

Regular Exercise: Engage in regular low-impact exercises such as swimming, walking, or gentle yoga to improve joint flexibility, strength, and overall physical function.

Physical Therapy: Work with a physical therapist to develop a personalized exercise program and learn techniques for joint protection, mobility, and pain management.

Joint Protection Techniques: Practice joint protection techniques such as using proper body mechanics, avoiding repetitive movements, and modifying activities to reduce joint stress and preserve function.

Adaptive Equipment: Consider using adaptive equipment such as jar openers, reachers, or kitchen gadgets with ergonomic handles to make daily tasks easier and reduce strain on joints.

C. BALANCING WORK, RELATIONSHIPS, AND SELF-CARE

Prioritize Self-Care: Make time for self-care activities such as adequate sleep, healthy eating, and stress management to support overall well-being and manage RA symptoms.

Set Realistic Goals: Set realistic goals for work, relationships, and daily activities, and be willing to adjust them based on your energy levels and pain levels.

Communicate with Others: Communicate openly with your employer, colleagues, family, and friends about your RA and any limitations or accommodations you may need. Educate them about the impact of RA on your daily life.

Seek Support: Lean on your support network for emotional and practical support. Joining support groups or connecting with others who have RA can provide valuable encouragement, understanding, and coping strategies.

D. TIPS FOR COMMUNICATING WITH HEALTHCARE PROVIDERS

Be Prepared: Before your appointment, write down any questions or concerns you have about your RA symptoms, treatment, or medication side effects.

Be Honest: Be honest with your healthcare provider about your symptoms, pain levels, and how RA is affecting your daily life. This information helps them make informed decisions about your treatment plan.

Ask for Clarification: If you don't understand something your healthcare provider says, don't hesitate to ask for clarification or additional information.

Be Proactive: Take an active role in your healthcare by advocating for yourself and expressing your preferences and goals for treatment. Collaborate with your healthcare provider to develop a personalized treatment plan that meets your needs and lifestyle.

CHAPTER FOUR

EMPOWERING YOURSELF AGAINST RHEUMATOID ARTHRITIS

A. Advocating For Your Needs: Tips For Self-Advocacy

B. Building A Support Network

C. Engaging In Research And Clinical Trials

D. Hope For The Future: Advances In Ra Treatment

A. ADVOCATING FOR YOUR NEEDS: TIPS FOR SELF-ADVOCACY

Educate Yourself: Learn as much as you can about RA, including its causes, symptoms, treatments, and available resources. Knowledge empowers you to make informed decisions about your care.

Communicate Effectively: Clearly communicate your needs, concerns, and treatment goals with your healthcare providers. Be assertive and advocate for yourself to ensure your voice is heard during medical appointments and treatment discussions.

Seek Second Opinions: If you're unsure about a diagnosis or treatment plan, don't hesitate to seek a second opinion from another healthcare provider. It's important to feel confident and comfortable with your treatment decisions.

Access Resources: Explore available resources such as patient advocacy organizations, support groups, online forums, and educational materials to connect with others living with RA and access additional support and information.

B. BUILDING A SUPPORT NETWORK

Family and Friends: Lean on your family and friends for emotional support, practical assistance, and companionship. Share your experiences with them and let them know how they can support you.

Support Groups: Joining a support group for individuals with RA can provide valuable emotional support, encouragement, and practical advice from others who understand what you're going through.

Online Communities: Participate in online communities and forums for people with RA to connect with others, share experiences, and exchange information and tips for managing the condition.

Professional Support: Consider seeking support from a therapist or counselor who specializes in chronic illness or pain management to help you cope with the emotional challenges of living with RA.

C. ENGAGING IN RESEARCH AND CLINICAL TRIALS

Stay Informed: Stay updated on the latest research and advancements in RA treatment by following reputable sources such as medical journals, patient advocacy organizations, and healthcare websites.

Consider Clinical Trials: Talk to your healthcare provider about whether participating in a clinical trial for RA treatment is a viable option for you. Clinical trials offer access to cutting-edge treatments and contribute to the advancement of medical knowledge.

Ask Questions: If you're considering participating in a clinical trial, ask your healthcare provider about the potential risks and benefits, eligibility criteria, and what participation entails.

D. HOPE FOR THE FUTURE: ADVANCES IN RA TREATMENT

Biologic Therapies: Advances in biologic therapies have revolutionized the treatment of RA, offering targeted approaches to suppress inflammation and slow down joint damage. New biologic agents continue to be developed and researched, providing hope for improved outcomes and quality of life for individuals with RA.

Precision Medicine: Research into personalized or precision medicine approaches aims to tailor treatment plans to individual patients based on their unique genetic, environmental, and clinical characteristics. This personalized approach holds promise for optimizing treatment effectiveness and minimizing side effects in RA management.

Novel Therapies: Ongoing research is exploring novel therapeutic targets and treatment modalities for RA, including small molecule inhibitors, gene therapy, and regenerative medicine approaches. These innovative treatments have the potential to offer new options for individuals with RA who do not respond adequately to existing therapies.

Multidisciplinary Care: The integration of multidisciplinary care teams, including rheumatologists, physical therapists, occupational therapists, and mental health professionals, can provide comprehensive and holistic management of RA, addressing not only the physical symptoms but also the emotional and psychosocial aspects of the disease. This collaborative approach offers hope for better outcomes and improved quality of life for individuals living with RA.

Top of Form

SPECIAL CONSIDERATIONS

A. Ra And Women's Health

B. Ra In Children And Adolescents

C. Managing Ra In Older Adults

D. Ra And Comorbidities: Understanding The Connection

A. RA AND WOMEN'S HEALTH

Prevalence: Rheumatoid arthritis (RA) is more common in women than in men, with women being two to three times more likely to develop the condition. The reasons for this gender disparity are not fully understood but may involve hormonal factors, genetic predisposition, and differences in immune response.

Pregnancy: Pregnancy can have variable effects on RA symptoms. Some women experience improvement in symptoms during pregnancy, particularly in the second and third trimesters, while others may experience flares or worsening of symptoms. It's important for women with RA to work closely with their healthcare providers to manage their condition during pregnancy and ensure optimal outcomes for both mother and baby.

Menopause: Menopause can also impact RA symptoms, as hormonal changes during this time may affect disease activity. Some women may experience worsening of symptoms or increased disease activity after menopause. Hormone replacement therapy (HRT) may be considered in some cases, although its use in women with RA should be carefully evaluated based on individual risks and benefits.

B. RA IN CHILDREN AND ADOLESCENTS

Juvenile Idiopathic Arthritis (JIA): Rheumatoid arthritis that occurs in children and adolescents is referred to as juvenile idiopathic arthritis (JIA). JIA is the most common chronic rheumatic disease in childhood, affecting approximately 1 in 1,000 children.

Subtypes of JIA: JIA encompasses several subtypes, each with distinct clinical features and disease courses. These include oligoarticular JIA, polyarticular JIA, systemic-onset JIA, enthesitis-related arthritis, psoriatic arthritis, and undifferentiated arthritis.

Impact on Growth and Development: JIA can have significant effects on a child's physical growth, joint function, and psychosocial development. Early diagnosis and aggressive management are essential to prevent joint damage and disability.

Treatment Approaches: Treatment for JIA may involve a combination of medications (such as nonsteroidal anti-inflammatory drugs, disease-modifying antirheumatic drugs, and biologic agents), physical therapy, occupational therapy, and psychosocial support. The goal is to achieve disease remission, minimize symptoms, and promote optimal growth and development.

C. MANAGING RA IN OLDER ADULTS

Prevalence: While RA often develops in younger adults, it can also occur in older adults, including those over the age of 65. The prevalence of RA in older adults is increasing as the population ages.

Challenges in Diagnosis: RA in older adults may present differently than in younger populations, with atypical symptoms such as fatigue, weakness, and weight loss being more prominent. Additionally, comorbidities such as osteoarthritis, osteoporosis, and cardiovascular disease may complicate the diagnosis and management of RA in older adults.

Treatment Considerations: Treatment of RA in older adults should take into account age-related changes in physiology, comorbidities, and potential interactions with other medications. Nonpharmacological interventions, such as exercise, physical therapy, and assistive devices, may be particularly important in maintaining function and mobility in older adults with RA.

Balancing Risks and Benefits: Healthcare providers must carefully balance the risks and benefits of RA treatment in older adults, considering factors such as medication side effects, risk of falls and fractures, and overall functional status. Shared decision-making between patients and healthcare providers is essential to develop individualized treatment plans that optimize outcomes and quality of life.

D. RA AND COMORBIDITIES: UNDERSTANDING THE CONNECTION

Increased Risk of Comorbidities: Rheumatoid arthritis (RA) is associated with an increased risk of developing various comorbidities, including cardiovascular disease, osteoporosis, infections, lung disease, and psychological disorders such as depression and anxiety.

Shared Risk Factors: RA and its comorbidities share common risk factors such as inflammation, immune dysregulation, genetic predisposition, and lifestyle factors (e.g., smoking, sedentary lifestyle, unhealthy diet). Chronic inflammation in RA contributes to the development and progression of comorbidities through systemic effects on multiple organ systems.

Impact on Disease Management: Comorbidities can complicate the management of RA by affecting treatment choices, disease activity, and overall prognosis. For example, cardiovascular disease is a leading cause of mortality in individuals with RA, highlighting the importance of addressing cardiovascular risk factors and implementing preventive measures.

Integrated Approach to Care: Managing RA and its comorbidities requires an integrated, multidisciplinary approach that addresses both rheumatologic and non-rheumatologic aspects of care. Close collaboration between rheumatologists, primary care providers, specialists, and allied health professionals is essential to optimize outcomes and reduce the burden of comorbidities in individuals with RA. Regular monitoring, preventive screenings, and lifestyle interventions are key components of comprehensive RA management.

BEYOND THE INDIVIDUAL: RA IN SOCIETY

A. The Socioeconomic Impact Of Ra

B. Accessibility And Equity In Ra Care

C. Advocacy Efforts And Policy Changes

D. Promoting Awareness And Education

A. THE SOCIOECONOMIC IMPACT OF RA

Work Disability: RA can significantly impact an individual's ability to work, leading to absenteeism, presenteeism (reduced productivity while at work), and, in some cases, permanent disability. This can result in financial strain for individuals and their families and loss of productivity for employers.

Healthcare Costs: The direct and indirect costs associated with RA, including medical expenses, medications, rehabilitation, and lost productivity, impose a substantial economic burden on healthcare systems, governments, and society as a whole.

Impact on Quality of Life: RA can affect various aspects of quality of life, including physical functioning, mental health, social relationships, and overall well-being. The chronic nature of the disease and its associated symptoms can lead to decreased quality of life and increased healthcare utilization.

B. ACCESSIBILITY AND EQUITY IN RA CARE

Healthcare Disparities: Access to timely diagnosis, specialized care, and effective treatment for RA may be limited for certain populations, including racial and ethnic minorities, low-income individuals, and those living in rural or underserved areas. Healthcare disparities can exacerbate existing inequities in RA outcomes and exacerbate health disparities.

Barriers to Care: Barriers to accessing RA care may include financial barriers (e.g., lack of health insurance, high out-of-pocket costs), geographical barriers (e.g., limited access to rheumatologists or specialized care facilities), and cultural or linguistic barriers (e.g., language barriers, cultural beliefs about illness and treatment).

Promoting Equity: Efforts to promote equity in RA care involve addressing systemic barriers to access, advocating for policies that improve access to care for underserved populations, increasing cultural competence and diversity in healthcare providers, and ensuring that healthcare services are responsive to the needs of diverse communities.

C. ADVOCACY EFFORTS AND POLICY CHANGES

Patient Advocacy Organizations: Patient advocacy organizations play a crucial role in raising awareness about RA, advocating for the needs of individuals living with RA, and promoting policy changes to improve access to care, research funding, and quality of life for patients.

Policy Changes: Policy changes at the local, national, and international levels can have a significant impact on RA care and outcomes. This may include policies related to healthcare financing, insurance coverage, disability rights, workplace accommodations, and research funding.

Collaborative Efforts: Collaboration between patient advocacy organizations, healthcare providers, researchers, policymakers, and other stakeholders is essential for driving systemic change and addressing the complex challenges faced by individuals with RA in society.

D. PROMOTING AWARENESS AND EDUCATION

Public Awareness Campaigns: Public awareness campaigns can help increase understanding of RA among the general public, reduce stigma, and promote early detection and intervention. These campaigns may include educational materials, social media campaigns, community events, and media outreach.

Health Education Programs: Health education programs targeted at individuals living with RA, their families, caregivers, and healthcare providers can provide valuable information about the disease, treatment options, self-management strategies, and resources for support.

Community Engagement: Engaging with local communities, schools, workplaces, and healthcare settings can help raise awareness about RA and foster a supportive environment for individuals living with the condition. This may involve hosting informational sessions, support groups, or advocacy events.

CONCLUSION

A. Recap Of Key Points

B. Encouragement And Inspiration For Readers

C. Call To Action: Taking Charge Of Your Ra Journey

D. Looking Ahead: Hope For A Future Without Rheumatoid Arthritis

A. RECAP OF KEY POINTS

In this comprehensive exploration of rheumatoid arthritis (RA), we've covered a wide range of topics:

We discussed the definition, causes, and pathophysiology of RA, highlighting its autoimmune nature and its impact on joints and other systems in the body.

We examined the importance of addressing RA in modern society, considering its prevalence, economic burden, and public health implications.

We explored the various aspects of living with RA, including coping strategies, lifestyle modifications, treatment options, and the importance of self-advocacy.

We delved into special considerations such as RA's impact on women's health, children and adolescents, older adults, and its connection to comorbidities.

We considered the broader societal implications of RA, including its socioeconomic impact, accessibility and equity in care, advocacy efforts, and the importance of promoting awareness and education.

B. ENCOURAGEMENT AND INSPIRATION FOR READERS

Living with RA can be challenging, but it's important to remember that you're not alone in your journey. You have the strength and resilience to navigate the ups and downs of RA and to overcome the obstacles that may come your way. You are more than your diagnosis, and your experiences with RA can make you stronger, more compassionate, and more determined to live life to the fullest. Take comfort in the support of your loved ones, healthcare providers, and the broader RA community, and never underestimate the power of hope, positivity, and perseverance.

C. CALL TO ACTION: TAKING CHARGE OF YOUR RA JOURNEY

As you continue your RA journey, remember that you have the ability to take charge of your health and well-being. Be proactive in managing your condition by staying informed, advocating for your needs, and actively participating in your treatment plan. Prioritize self-care, listen to your body, and don't hesitate to reach out for support when you need it. Empower yourself to make informed decisions about your care, and remember that you are the most important advocate for your health.

D. LOOKING AHEAD: HOPE FOR A FUTURE WITHOUT RHEUMATOID ARTHRITIS

While living with RA can present challenges, there is hope for a future without rheumatoid arthritis. Ongoing research into the underlying causes of RA, advances in treatment options, and efforts to promote early detection and intervention offer promise for improved outcomes and quality of life for individuals affected by RA. By working together to raise awareness, advocate for policy changes, and support research efforts, we can move closer to a future where rheumatoid arthritis is better understood, effectively managed, and ultimately prevented. Together, let's envision a world where individuals with RA can live their lives free from the burden of this debilitating disease.

THE END

www.ingramcontent.com/pod-product-compliance
Lightning Source LLC
Chambersburg PA
CBHW050014230526
45470CB00003B/966